Low Carb Diet For Weight Loss Secrets

How To Effortlessly Lose Weight Fast With The Low Carb Diet

&

Low Carb Recipes for Weight Loss

50 Delicious Recipes to Effortlessly Lose Weight Fast

©Copyright 2015 by Matthew Jones - All rights reserved.

This document is geared towards providing exact and reliable information in regards to the topic and issue covered. The publication is sold with the idea that the publisher is not required to render accounting, officially permitted, or otherwise, qualified services. If advice is necessary, legal or professional, a practiced individual in the profession should be ordered.

- From a Declaration of Principles which was accepted and approved equally by a Committee of the American Bar Association and a Committee of Publishers and Associations.

In no way is it legal to reproduce, duplicate, or transmit any part of this document in either electronic means or in printed format. Recording of this publication is strictly prohibited and any storage of this document is not allowed unless with written permission from the publisher. All rights reserved.

The information provided herein is stated to be truthful and consistent, in that any liability, in terms of inattention or otherwise, by any usage or abuse of any policies, processes, or directions contained within is the solitary and utter responsibility of the recipient reader. Under no circumstances will any legal responsibility or blame be held against the publisher for any reparation, damages, or monetary loss due to the information herein, either directly or indirectly.

Respective authors own all copyrights not held by the publisher.

The information herein is offered for informational purposes solely, and is universal as so. The presentation of the information is without contract or any type of guarantee assurance.

The trademarks that are used are without any consent, and the publication of the trademark is without permission or backing by the trademark owner. All trademarks and brands within this book are for clarifying purposes only and are the owned by the owners themselves, not affiliated with this document.

TABLE OF CONTENTS

Low Carb Diet For Weight Loss Secrets 1
How To Effortlessly Lose Weight Fast With The Low Carb Diet 1

Introduction 1
What Is The Low Carb Diet? 2
Does It Work? 3
Top 5 Weight Loss Secrets 4
Successful Strategies To Implement The Low Carb Diet In Your Life 7
    Would You Describe Yourself As Addicted To Unhealthy Food? 7
    Do You Have Problems With Your Willpower And Self-Discipline? 8
    Are You A More Imaginative Person? 9
Effortless Weight Loss 10
Low Carb Diet Tips And Suggestions 13
Getting From Thinking And Planning To Doing 15
Low Carb Diet Recipes To Get You Started 17
Conclusion 32

Low Carb Recipes for Weight Loss
50 Delicious Recipes to Effortlessly Lose Weight Fast

Introduction 34
Chapter 1 - 10 Low Carb Breakfast Recipes 35
Chapter 2 - 10 Low Carb Lunch and Dinner Recipes 45
Chapter 3 - 10 Low Carb Side Dish Recipes 55
Chapter 4 - 10 Low Carb Snack Recipes 64
Chapter 5 - 10 Low Carb Dessert Recipes 75
Conclusion 85

INTRODUCTION

I want to thank you and congratulate you for buying the book, *"Low Carb Diet For Weight Loss Secrets-How To Effortlessly Lose Weight With The Low Carb Diet"*.

This book expounds on the low carb diet and introduces several weight loss secrets as well as strategies and tips on how to successfully implement the low carb diet in your life.

There is a high chance that you've already tried a ton of different diet plans and weight loss strategies that simply didn't lead to the desired weight loss effect, or you just lost the weight only to gain it all back. Chances are you've tried your best, but the techniques simply didn't work. If this is the case, you don't have to worry. This book will not only give you the information you need to know about the low carb diet and its amazing benefits but also provide you with a few easy strategies and tips on how to effortlessly get rid of the few excess pounds.

You will be happy to know, that the low carb diet is quite different from other diets. It has been proven by various scientific sources that the low carb diet is extremely beneficial to your health. However, this is not even the best part. What's great about the low carb diet is that it requires little to no excess work. Don't think that there aren't challenges that arise from the implementation of the low carb diet. As with any other diet or life-changing plan, you will have to face certain restrictions, which may be a bit too much for your willpower. However, this book will provide you with a few low carb diet weight loss secrets, tips and strategies to help you easily deal with any challenge that arises from the restrictions of the diet.

WHAT IS THE LOW CARB DIET?

If you have chosen the low carb diet, you are already on the right path to effortless weight loss. The low carb diet is not only a great way to get rid of the excess pounds, but also has many health benefits. However, what exactly is the low carb diet?

Carbohydrates in food are the prime source of energy for our bodies. They perform numerous roles in our bodies, including the storage of energy, improving our immune system and more. They are an important part of our nutrition, but are also the prime factor for excess fat and obesity. Why?

Most of the foods that we love to eat have high quantities of carbohydrates. While it is important for our body to have energy, we only manage to use a small portion of the energy that we get from the carbohydrates. The rest of the energy is conserved in the body in form of fat.

The low carb diet is concentrated on lowering carbohydrate intake, without you having to face a lot of restrictions and challenges. Generally used to lose weight effortlessly, the diet has several health benefits. For instance, it reduces the risk factors associated with diabetes, cancer, heart disease and more.

Moreover, as there are only a few challenges that you will have to face if you implement the low crab diet in your life, you will not only be getting slimmer, but will also be:

i. Enjoying various amounts of different foods.

ii. Changing Your Eating Habits for the Better.

iii. Strengthening your Immune System.

DOES IT WORK?

As aforementioned, carbohydrates are our bodies' main source of fuel. Carbohydrates are classified into two categories namely sugars and starches, which fuel every activity you are involved in. It seems unnatural that lowering your carbohydrate intake, as the low carb diet suggests, will help you lose weight while gaining health benefits. However, it is true.

When our carbohydrate intake is too high, most of the carbohydrates in our body are directly converted into excess fat. They also trigger the production of more insulin, the fat storing hormone. The more carbohydrates are in your body, the more glucose is in your blood thus the more insulin is produced. This leads to serious diseases such as heart disease and diabetes and prevents the fat breakdown in your body.

The low carb diet truly does works. However, what is best about it is that you have one of the widest varieties of foods available for you to eat. Therefore, if you don't like monotonous meals every day, you will love the low carb diet. As with any diet, there are restrictions and you will have to face certain challenges that will test your will power. The fact still remains that the low carb diet is definitely one of the easiest and effortless ways to achieve weight loss.

TOP 5 WEIGHT LOSS SECRETS

Before delving more into the low carb diet, it would be important for you to know some weight loss secrets that will make it easier for you to face the challenges that come with adopting any diet including the low carb diet.

Secret #1: Exercise Is Great and Does Not Always Require Effort

Even though the low carb diet will help you get rid of your excess pounds rather quickly, the process still needs time. However, if you combine the diet with regular exercise, you will be able to see results much more quickly. One of the things you should be aware of is that exercise does not always require effort. If you have no time or simply do not want to go to the gym or jog in the park, don't worry; there is a ton of other ways to get your body to burn fat. One of the best ways is through yoga, Pilates or dancing. But you know what's even better? Sex! That's right; don't be scared to get frisky, as it will help you get rid of excess fat even faster.

Secret #2: Dieting Can be Rather Fun

What most people don't take into account is the positive sides of diets that come on top of the health benefits and the weight loss. When talking about the low carb diet, you'd be surprised by the variety of foods available that you did not even know existed simply by concentrating more on your carbohydrates. Start this diet with the enthusiasm that you will get to eat new foods and tasty meals without necessarily having to take carbohydrates.

Secret #3: It's All About the Mindset

It is scientifically proven that your mindset has an effect on your performance when starting any action. If you think of the diet as a positive new thing for you, then you will have no problem with starting the low carb diet. Moreover, if you keep your mindset about the diet in the positive scale, you will be seeing the weight loss benefits much faster.

Secret #4: Get your Sleep Schedule Right

One of the most important factors that are overlooked by many is sleep. Although, people don't tend to stress on the importance of a healthy sleep schedule in diets, sleep is a vital part of your weight loss even when you talk of the essence of exercise. Sleep helps the body regenerate, while keeping everything in check. If you want your diet to be successful, get enough sleep.

Secret #5: Be Careful Who You Tell

Have you tried dieting before? Have you told the people who are closest to you what you will be doing? Did they make jokes? If the answer is yes, don't worry. It is common that the people who are closest to you will make jokes and statements regarding your success or failure. It is almost certain that they don't want to harm you in any way, but the truth is, they do. Each statement or a joke has a negative impact on both your conscious and subconscious mind. Make sure not to tell many people when dieting, as it will definitely be easier for you if you keep it to yourself at first. Share with people your plan once you feel confident enough that you are going to succeed with it. Telling people who are likely to support you will also give you the morale to go on. Actually, you will have a stronger drive since you will not want to let down these people.

SUCCESSFUL STRATEGIES TO IMPLEMENT THE LOW CARB DIET IN YOUR LIFE

As mentioned in the previous chapter, you need to be aware of different weight loss secrets when going on a low carb diet. However, knowing that you want to go on a low carb diet and actually doing it are completely different things. Here are a few basic successful strategies you can use based on your character description in order to implement the low carb diet in your life easily.

Would You Describe Yourself As Addicted To Unhealthy Food?

One of the worst cases is when you want to implement a diet in your life when you are addicted to unhealthy food. If this is the case for you, make sure to concentrate on your willpower as much as possible. However, don't stress out and don't worry. The easiest way to get rid of an addiction is to replace it with another good habit; something you equally love but is not harmful.

Just as smokers quit cigarettes by chewing gum, try to replace your addiction to unhealthy food with a healthy one. This may seem impossible, but it is far easier to do. Once you have chosen to implement the low carb diet in your life, you will have a ton of tasty options of food to choose from. Every time you think of unhealthy food, simply head to the cupboard and get some almonds or drink a glass of water until you feel that your hunger is tamed.

This strategy works well in taming food addiction. Remember, you are not addicted to the unhealthy food as much as you are addicted to the habit of eating it. If you replace the habit with eating more healthy food, it will be far easier to you to implement the low carb diet in your life.

Do You Have Problems With Your Willpower And Self-Discipline?

If you experience more trouble with your willpower and the self-discipline part of the implementation of the diet rather than the food itself, you can try implementing different tips and tricks that will help you out on your path to successful weight loss.

One of the best tips, as mentioned before is keeping a positive mindset. Rather than perceiving the diet as something that you "must" or "have to" do, choose to view it as something that you "choose to" do. Make sure to always have conversations with yourself. Even though this may sound far-fetched, it is extremely helpful.

For example, every time you hear your inner voice telling you that you "can't continue" doing the diet. Ask yourself "why?" Ask yourself further questions, such as "why did I choose to undertake this diet in the first place?" Self-talk is helpful regarding any issue connected with self-discipline and is an extremely helpful strategy to keep in mind when implementing the low carb diet.

Another thing you might try is to separate your food and snacks in portions. Make sure to keep a few portions of your meal, the portions being not bigger than two of your fists, in your fridge. Separate your snacks into portions as well. When starting to eat, take one of the portions. When finished eating, even if you go to the fridge for a second one, you will most probably never go for a third. This will help you out a lot, as you will be able to have more time to talk and ask yourself the valuable questions, when going to get that next meal. This will help you eat relatively less than you usually do; you will be surprised as to how helpful it actually is.

Are You A More Imaginative Person?

If you describe yourself as an imaginative person, then make sure to use this to your advantage when implementing the low carb diet. Your mindset is truly a powerful thing and if you are quite imaginative, you should always try to visualize the diet as something amazing. Whether you will envision the diet as a fun new experience or a vicious challenge that you have to complete in order for you to be a better person is totally up to you. However, make sure that the said vision of the diet will be most beneficial to you.

EFFORTLESS WEIGHT LOSS

After you've familiarized yourself with the basics of the low carb diet and the successful strategies, secrets and tips that you have to know in order to successfully implement the diet in your life, it is time to learn why it is effortless. The answer to the question is rather simple – the diet requires little to no effort because you have a wide variety of foods to eat. How exactly do you choose your food and which foods you should avoid? Which are the most common foods with high quantities of carbohydrates?

The basic foods that you shall eat include:

- Meat
- Fish
- Eggs
- Vegetables
- Fruits
- Nuts
- Seeds
- High-Fat Dairy
- Healthy Fats & Oils
- The basic foods that you shall not eat include:
- Sugar
- Wheat
- Seed Oils

- Artificial Sweeteners
- Low-Fat Products
- Highly Processed "Diet" and Low-Fat Food

The general consumption of sugar is probably the most difficult to avoid, but if you implement the strategies mentioned in the previous chapters in the book, you will find it far easier to start your low carb diet.

Need a more detailed list of foods to avoid? Here's a quick one:

Sugar is contained in many things, but you most generally should avoid fruit juices, agave, ice cream, cakes, soft drinks, and many others.

Gluten Grains: Any type of bread, wheat products, spelt, pastas and more.

"Low-Fat" Products: Generally, any product that is labeled as "diet" or "low-fat" is highly processed; thus, it is very unhealthy for you to eat especially due to its high carbohydrate quantities

Other Highly Processed Foods: Anything that is processed is not recommended

High Omega-6-Seed and Vegetable oils: Though oils are considered good in some cases, any vegetable oil should be avoided in the low carb diet

Trans Fats: Especially "Hydrogenated" or "partially hydrogenated" oils should also be avoided.

As you have noticed, you don't have to avoid that many food choices. Probably, the hardest one to avoid is the sugar, as it is found in almost everything. However, make sure to give it your best to avoid it in order to achieve fast and effortless weight loss via the low carb diet. You may consider using honey or any other natural sweetener that may not contain as much calories (this should definitely controlled).

If you want to be more exact in the numbers as to what your carbohydrate intake should be, make sure to focus to a maximum of 50 to 150 grams per day. However, be sure to aim at more healthy carbohydrate choices and avoid sugars.

LOW CARB DIET TIPS AND SUGGESTIONS

By now, you should be familiar with almost everything needed for you to implement the low carb diet in your life. However, it is not always as easy as it sounds. For some, the "all or nothing" approach may be beneficial, but in most cases, people fail after the first few weeks or even days. If you want to truly succeed,

you should be in for the long haul.

Start making small changes in your diet. For example, in the first few days, change only one of your meals to be a low carb one then go with two and after two-three weeks, make sure to follow the rules of the low carb diet fully. This does not grant an instant result, but it is an effortless weight loss method. Additionally, this will definitely change your eating habits for the better.

Keeping track of your progress is also an essential part of the low carb diet. Once you have replaced all of your meals with low carb meals, make sure to start keeping track of your progress. However, don't only trust the scale and what it shows. Make sure to take regular pictures of your body every week for your own personal assessment. Usually, the first results of the low carb diet can be noticed within three weeks of the official start of your low carb diet.

The first month of the diet is the hardest mainly because the results are not visibly noticeable. However, once you reach the one-month mark, be rest assured that you will visibly be getting thinner every single week. Make sure to keep your positive mindset at all times.

Even if you 'fail' midway the diet by eating something that you should avoid, don't quit and mark that as a failure, but rather continue with the diet. One of the biggest mistakes you can make is to consider your diet a failure when you eat one meal that is not included in the diet plan. However, you may tend to slack off a bit. That being said, one meal out of the diet every now and then won't be a huge issue but you should always try to avoid it. Make sure not to give yourself excuses but rather act more, keep a positive mindset and remind yourself why and how the low carb diet will help you out.

Another common mistake you can make when on a low carb diet is to think that a healthy eating habit requires a big budget. This is not necessarily the case with the low carb diet. What I love more about the low carb diet is that you will actually be spending less money for food, which is far healthier for you and will lead you to effortless weight loss.

GETTING FROM THINKING AND PLANNING TO DOING

Once you have created a diet plan like the one given in the chapter above, you should get from thinking and planning to actually doing. This is the most important part of the process and a point at which many people fail. Once you are ready to start, don't give yourself excuses and just get going. Rather than setting a date, or a day of the month, simply start the change today. You will see that once you start, everything becomes far easier.

At this point, you should already be ready mentally to start your diet. All you have to do is act. If you don't have the time to create a detailed meal plan, don't worry. Just make sure that you get rid of all food that you should avoid and buy food that you should eat in the low carb diet.

It may sound extreme, but if you are ready to start the diet and are confident in yourself, simply get up and clean your fridge and cupboards from everything that you should avoid. Give it to a friend or a neighbor, because if there is no such food within your reach, the chances that you will fail in your diet are greatly reduced. We are all human and at the end of the day, when something is right in front of us, regardless of our willpower, we may not be able to avoid it. So make sure to get rid of food that you should avoid. Go to the market and buy food that you truly need to implement into your diet plan.

Don't know what exactly to buy? Here's a short list of items:

- Eggs
- Cottage Cheese
- Tuna (without additional oils)

- Any fruits or vegetables that you like
- Soybeans
- Meat (Chicken, beef, fish)
- Turkey slices
- Dressings and Spices (such as the fat free thousand island dressing)
- Crackers
- Almonds
- Any Type of Nuts

Once your home is full of low carb food, it will be far easier for you to actually implement your diet. Beware, as the first two weeks are probably the most important ones in your path to weight loss. However, once you get in the habit of eating right, you will be left surprised as to how easy it actually is to lose weight and have the lean body that you've always wanted.

Give yourself time and don't be stressed. Big changes in your life require time and nothing can happen in an instant. However, every day you will be getting closer and closer to a change for the better. Once again, make sure to keep that in mind and remind yourself why you have chosen the low carb diet.

LOW CARB DIET RECIPES TO GET YOU STARTED

This book would not be complete without a few recipes to get you started on your journey to losing weight with the low carb diet. Below are several recipes you can try out.

Low Carb Breakfast recipes

Almond Strawberry smoothie

Ingredients

16 oz. unsweetened almond milk

¼ cup frozen strawberries

4 oz. heavy cream

1 tsp vanilla extract

½ tsp artificial sweetener

Instructions

Put all ingredients in your blender and blend until smooth. Add a little water to thin it down.

Serves 1.

Low Carb Breakfast Meatballs

Ingredients

1 lb lean ground beef

2 tbsp onion, minced

32 oz. pork sausage

½ lb shredded cheddar cheese

Ground black pepper to taste

3 eggs

Instructions

Preheat oven to 350° F.

Combine all ingredients in a bowl and mix thoroughly. Roll into 1 ½" balls and place on a baking sheet. Bake for 18-20 minutes.

This makes around fifty to sixty meatballs.

Serves 15.

Broccoli and Cheese Quiche

Ingredients

10 oz. broccoli

¾ cup shredded mozzarella cheese

3 slices of lean ham

5 eggs

1 cup of sliced mushrooms

Instructions

Spray a pan with cooking spray.

Layer the pan with mushrooms, chopped broccoli, cheese and ham.

Beat eggs with water then pour in pan.

Bake at 350° F for twenty minutes.

Serves 6.

Egg Crepes

Ingredients

2 eggs

2 tbsp heavy cream

Instructions

Blend the ingredients in a blender.

Heat a pan with some oil.

Pour the mixture in the pan and as it starts to come away from the edges, turn carefully with a spatula. Slide the crepe onto a place until the mixture is finished.

Season with cinnamon and artificial sweetener.

Serves 1.

Hash Brown Potato Cakes

Ingredients

1 lb round red potatoes

1 tbsp olive oil

½ onion, thinly sliced

¼ tsp salt

2 tsp fresh thyme

Nonstick cooking spray

1/8 tsp black pepper, ground

Instructions

Preheat oven to 300 degrees F. Peel and shred potatoes, rinse with cold water, drain well, pressing lightly then pat dry with paper towels and put in a large bowl. Stir onion, thyme, salt, oil, and pepper into the potatoes.

Coat a nonstick saucepan with cooking spray. Preheat the skillet over medium-high heat. For every cake, scoop a tablespoon of the potato mixture onto the skillet. Press down the potato mixture with a spatula to flatten evenly. Cook for five minutes then turn the potatoes and cook for another five minutes or until golden brown.

Place the cooked potatoes on a baking sheet. Keep them warm and uncovered in the oven as you cook the remaining potato cakes.

Serves 8.

Low carb Main dishes

Steak with garlic butter

Ingredients

4 lb beef sirloin steak

2 tsp garlic powder

½-cup butter

4 cloves garlic, minced

Black pepper and salt to taste

Instructions

Prepare an outdoor grill for high heat.

In a small pan, over medium heat, melt the butter and cook the garlic then set aside.

Grill the steaks for five minutes each side. Once done, transfer to warmed plates and brush the tops with the garlic butter. Allow to rest for around two minutes before serving.

Serves 8.

Chicken breasts stuffed with spinach

Ingredients

4 skinless, boneless chicken breasts

1 10 oz. package chopped spinach, thawed and drained

2 cloves garlic, chopped

½ cup crumbled feta cheese

½ cup mayonnaise

4 slices of bacon

Instructions

Preheat oven to 375 degrees F.

Mix the mayonnaise, feta cheese, spinach and garlic until well blended then put aside.

Butterfly the chicken wings ensuring not to cut all the way through.

Spoon the spinach mixture into the chicken breasts and wrap

each with a piece of bacon then secure using a toothpick. Put in a shallow baking dish and cover.

Bake for one hour or until the chicken is no longer pink.

Serves 4.

Braised Balsamic Chicken

Ingredients

6 skinless, boneless chicken breast halves

½ cup balsamic vinegar

2 tbsp olive oil

1 tsp garlic salt

1 onion, sliced

Ground black pepper to taste

½ tsp dried thyme

1 cup of diced tomatoes

1 tsp dried oregano

1 tsp dried basil

1 tsp dried rosemary

Instructions

Season the chicken with the garlic salt and pepper.

Heat oil in a pan over medium heat, cook the chicken until browned for around three to four minutes each side. Add the onions and cook until the onions have browned.

Pour the diced tomatoes and the vinegar over the chicken, season with oregano, thyme, rosemary and basil. Simmer the chicken for twenty-five minutes or until the juices run clear. This should be around 15 minutes.

Serves 6.

Honey Mustard Pork burgers

Ingredients

1 lb ground pork breakfast sausage

1 egg white, whisked

1 cup plantain chips

1 garlic clove, minced

3 tbsp bacon fat

1/2tsp garlic powder

Black pepper and salt to taste

1 tbsp raw honey

1 avocado, sliced

1 tsp yellow mustard

1 tsp Dijon mustard

Arugula to garnish

Instructions

Preheat the oven to 350 degrees F.

Put the plantain chips in the food processor and pulse until broken down into breadcrumb consistency.

Place the egg white in one bowl and the plantain crumbs in another. Dip each burger patty in the egg whites then plantain mixture to coat burgers completely then sprinkle with salt, garlic powder and pepper.

Heat a cast iron skillet over medium high heat, place two tbsp of bacon fat in the skillet and add the minced garlic.

Immediately the garlic becomes fragrant, add the pork burgers to the pan and cook both sides for four minutes.

Once the burgers are cooked on each side, place in the oven and cook for ten minutes. .

Whisk together the mustards, honey, and slice up the avocado.

Remove the burgers from the oven and allow them to rest for three minutes to prevent the juices from coming out.

Top each burger with the avocado and honey mustard.

Serves 4.

Herb crusted Salmon

Ingredients

2 salmon fillets

2 tbsp fresh parsley

1 tbsp coconut flour

1 tbsp Dijon mustard

2 tbsp olive oil

2 cups arugula

Juice of 1 lemon

¼ red onion, sliced

1 tbsp white wine vinegar

Black pepper and salt to taste

Instructions

Preheat oven to 450 degrees F.

Place the salmon on a baking sheet lined with foil.

Top the salmon with Dijon mustard and 1 tablespoon olive oil and rub into the salmon.

Mix the coconut flour, salt, pepper and parsley.

Sprinkle the toppings on the salmon then pat into the salmon using your hand.

Place in the oven for ten to 15 minutes.

While the salmon is cooking, mix the arugula, onion, lemon juice, salt, pepper, white wine vinegar and 1 tablespoon of olive oil.

Once cooked, top the salmon with the salad.

Low carb soups and salads

Bacon and Chicken Soup

Ingredients

12 slices bacon

10 oz. boneless skinless cooked chicken breasts

1 onion, diced

1 cup heavy whipping cream

1 bell pepper, chopped

1 cup chicken broth

1 1/3 cup Mexican shredded cheese

10 oz. cream cheese

8 celery stalks

1 yellow squash

1 small zucchini squash

8 cups of water

Instructions

Allow the water to boil and add any seasonings you want.

Chop all vegetables and add to the pot then reduce heat and allow to simmer.

Fry the bacon until crisp and set aside.

Chop the chicken into cubes, fry until crisp and put aside. Crunch the bacon into small pieces.

Add the chicken broth and cream. Simmer for twenty minutes.

Serve and top with Mexican cheese, bacon and cream cheese.

Tomato soup

Ingredients

28 ounce can diced tomatoes, undrained

2 cups chicken, broth

½ cup onion

2 tbsp butter

1 cup heavy cream

2 tbsp parsley, minced

Black pepper and salt to taste

Instructions

Sauté onion in butter until tender. Add the tomatoes with their liquid and broth then bring to a boil. Simmer for five minutes. Puree using a stick blender until you achieve a smooth consistency.

Stir in the cream and adjust the seasoning. Stir in the parsley and serve immediately.

Makes 6-8 servings or six cups.

Cream of Asparagus Soup

Ingredients

2 lb asparagus

2 tbsp low fat sour cream

6 cups fat free chicken broth

1 tbsp butter

1 medium onion, chopped

Salt and pepper to taste.

Instructions

Melt the butter on a large pot over low heat. Add onion and sauté on low heat for around 2 to 3 minutes.

Snap off the tough ends of the asparagus and discard. Chop the asparagus in two-inch pieces and add to the pot. Add the chicken broth, pepper and salt. Cover and cook for around 20-25 minutes.

Remove from the heat, add the sour cream, and puree until smooth using a hand held mixer.

Shrimp and Avocado Salad

Ingredients

Marinade

3 tbsp limejuice

½ cup chopped fresh cilantro

2 tbsp extra virgin olive oil

1/8 tsp fresh black pepper

Salt to taste

Salad

4 cups lettuce

2 ripe avocados

1 lb cooked shrimp, deveined and tail removed

Instructions

Pour the marinade over the shrimp, stir to coat and allow it to refrigerate for around an hour.

Wash and dry the lettuce and divide among plates.

Cut the avocado into wedges and sprinkle over the lettuce.

Top with the marinated shrimp and the leftover dressing.

Serves 4. If taken as dinner, serves 2.

Enchilada Chicken Avocado Salad

Ingredients

1 cup of leftover chicken

½ Avocado, diced

1 mango, peeled and diced

1 small head of hearts of romaine, shredded.

Instructions

Chop the romaine. Place the enchilada chicken on top.

Add the avocado and mongo on top of that.

Serves two.

Cucumber Salad

Ingredients

1 ½ English Cucumbers

1 tsp salt

2 tbsp cilantro, Chopped

4 large green onions

¼ cup fresh lemon juice

1 tsp lemon zest

¼ cup extra virgin olive oil

1/8 tsp freshly cracked pepper.

Instructions

Slice the cucumbers finely. Sprinkle with salt and allow them to sit on a colander in the sink for an hour.

Rinse the cucumbers thoroughly and let them drain on paper towels.

Slice green onions, chop the cilantro and zest the lemon. Combine these three with lemon juice, cracked pepper and olive oil.

Pour the dressing over the cucumber and mix thoroughly.

Apple Zucchini Crisp

Ingredients

1 cup of apples, peeled and sliced

2 cups of zucchini, peeled halved and sliced thinly

2 tsp cinnamon, divided

¼ cup splenda brown sugar

A pinch of nutmeg

3 tbsp lemon juice

1/3 cup sliced almonds

1/3 cup almond meal

1 tsp vanilla extract

1/3 cup chopped pecans

¼ cup butter melted

Instructions

Preheat oven to 375 degrees F.

Toss the zucchini, apples, lemon juice and one teaspoon of cinnamon powder.

Pour into a baking dish.

Mix the remaining one teaspoon of cinnamon, brown sugar, almond meal, nutmegs, pecans and almonds together.

Stir in the vanilla with melted butter and pour over the nut mixture while mixing thoroughly.

Crumble the nut mixture over the zucchini and apples.

Bake while uncovered for thirty minutes

Serves 8.

CONCLUSION

Thank you again for buying this book!

I hope this book was able to help you understand what the low carb diet is all about what to eat sparingly and what to avoid. This is the first step towards losing weight using the low carb diet. It is important that you start adopting the diet gradually so as not to overwhelm yourself which can lead to your eventual failure. You can start by substituting one of your meals with a low carb meal and overtime start changing your diet slowly with your goal to be to live a low carb diet lifestyle for permanent weight loss.

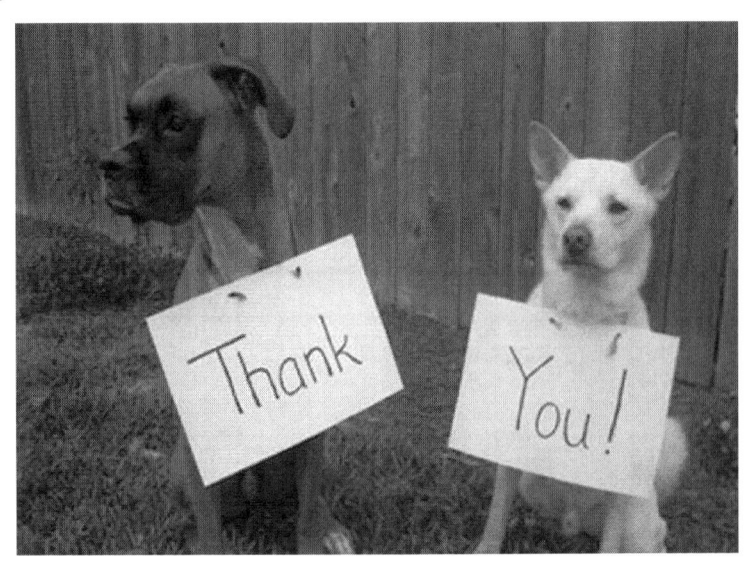

Finally, if you enjoyed this book, please take the time to share your thoughts and post a review on Amazon. It'd be greatly appreciated!

Thank you and good luck!

Low Carb Recipes for Weight Loss

50 Delicious Recipes to Effortlessly Lose Weight Fast

INTRODUCTION

I want to thank you and congratulate you for buying the book, "Low Carb Recipes for Weight Loss: 50 Delicious Recipes to Effortlessly Lose Weight Fast".

This book contains proven steps and strategies on how to make 50 delicious and easy to make low carb dishes at home.

In this book you will find 10 low carb recipes for each types of dishes: Breakfast, Main Course (for lunch and dinner), Sides, Snacks, and Desserts. Use these recipes to fill your meal plan and stick to it so that you can effortlessly lose weight!

Thanks again for buying this book, I hope you enjoy it!

CHAPTER 1

10 LOW CARB BREAKFAST RECIPES

Avocado and Ham Omelet

Makes: 2 servings

Ingredients:

- 4 Tbsp sour cream
- 4 eggs
- 1/2 cup minced ham
- 4 Tbsp diced tomato
- 1 avocado, cored, peeled and sliced
- Paprika
- Salt

Instructions:

1. Season the sour cream with salt and paprika. Beat the eggs with a fork.

2. Grease nonstick skillet and place over medium-high heat. To check

readiness, add a drop of water and watch if it sizzles. Pour the eggs into the skillet and tilt to spread evenly across the bottom.

3. Let the edges set then lift it and tilt to cook the runny part of the egg. Set heat on the lowest possible setting.

4. Add the tomato and ham. Put a lid on the skillet and set the heat on low. Cook for 1 minute or until top is set. Place the sliced avocado on top and fold the omelet. Spoon sour cream on top before serving.

Country Scrambled Eggs

Makes: 1 serving

Ingredients:

- 1/2 Tbsp butter
- 1/8 cup diced cooked ham
- 1/8 cup diced green pepper
- 2 eggs, beaten
- Salt
- Pepper

Instructions:

1. Place a skillet over medium heat and melt the butter. Saute the ham, green pepper, and onion until onion becomes soft.

2. Add the beaten eggs and scramble until set. Season with salt and pepper, and serve.

Gingerbread Waffles

Makes: 3 servings

Ingredients:

- 1/2 cup almond meal
- 1/2 cup vanilla whey protein powder
- 1/4 tsp salt
- 1/8 cup Splenda
- 1/2 Tbsp baking powder
- 1 tsp ground ginger
- 1/4 cup heavy cream
- 1/4 cup water
- 1 egg
- 2 Tbsp melted butter

Instructions:

1. Heat the waffle iron.

2. In a bowl, mix together the dry ingredients. Combine the cream and water in a glass measuring cup and then add the water and egg. Add the melted butter and mix well. Add this to the dry ingredients and stir to combine.

3. Pour some of the batter into the waffle iron and bake according to the manufacturer's instructions. Serve with whipped cream if preferred.

Hot Cinnamon Cereal

Makes: 2 to 3 servings

Ingredients:

- 1/2 cup ground flaxseeds
- 1/2 cup ground almonds
- 1/4 cup oat bran
- 3/4 cup wheat bran
- 1/4 cup vanilla flavored whey protein powder
- 1 tsp cinnamon

Instructions:

1. Mix the ingredients together in a bowl and keep in an airtight container.

2. To make one serving, scoop half a cup of the mixture into a bowl and add 3/4 cup boiling water. Add a pinch of salt and stir. Let sit for 2 to 3 minutes before eating.

French Toast

Makes: 3 servings

Ingredients:

- 2 eggs
- 1/4 cup heavy cream
- 1/4 cup water

Low Carb Recipes for Weight Loss

- 1/2 tsp vanilla
- 3 slices low carb bread of your choice
- Butter

Instructions:

1. Beat the eggs with the vanilla extract, heavy cream, and water. Put this in a shallow dish.

2. Soak each slice of bread in the mixture for 5 minutes, turning once.

3. Place a heavy skillet over medium heat and melt just enough butter to coat the base. Fry each piece of bread on both sides until brown.

4. Serve with sugar-free syrup, Splenda, and a sprinkle of cinnamon.

Low Carb Granola

Makes: 6 1/2 cups

Ingredients:

- 1 cup all-bran extra fiber cereal
- 1 1/2 cups shredded unsweetened coconut
- 1 cup rolled oats
- 1/2 cup pecan pieces
- 1/2 cup shelled raw pumpkin seeds
- 1/2 cup shelled raw sunflower seeds
- 12 cup sliced almonds

- 1/4 cup sesame seeds
- 1/2 cup ground flax seeds
- 1 1/2 Tbsp ground cinnamon
- 1/4 cup vanilla whey protein powder
- 1/2 tsp salt
- 1/2 cup melted butter
- 3/4 cup Splenda

Instructions:

1. Preheat oven to 350 degrees F (180 degrees C).

2. In a large mixing bowl, combine the dry ingredients.

3. In a separate bowl, combine the melted butter and Splenda. Mix well and pour this over the dry ingredients. Combine thoroughly.

4. Transfer the mixture into a baking pan and bake for 30 to 45 minutes or until lightly toasted. Make sure to stir every 15 minutes.

5. Set aside to cool to room temperature then store in a tightly sealed container.

Rice Bran and Flax Bread

Makes: approximately 22 slices

Ingredients:

- 2 cups and 4 Tbsp water
- 3/4 cup rice bran

Low Carb Recipes for Weight Loss

- 3/4 cup flaxseed meal
- 2 cups vital wheat gluten
- 3/4 cup vanilla flavored whey protein powder
- 4 tsp blackstrap molasses
- 2 tsp salt
- 2 Tbsp oil
- 4 tsp yeast

Instructions:

1. Pour all of the ingredients in a bread machine and process based on manufacturer's instructions.

2. Remove the loaf and set aside to cool.

Buttermilk Pancakes

Makes: 7 to 8 pancakes

Ingredients:

- 1/4 cup almond meal
- 1/4 cup vanilla whey protein powder
- 1/8 cup gluten
- 1 Tbsp wheat germ
- 1/2 Tbsp wheat bran
- 1/2 tsp baking powder

- 1/4 tsp baking soda
- 1/2 cup buttermilk
- 1 small egg
- 1 Tbsp melted butter

Instructions:

1. In a bowl, mix together the dry ingredients until well distributed.

2. In a glass measuring cup mix the egg, melted butter, and buttermilk. Stir to combine. Pour the mixture into the dry ingredients and stir with a whisk until completely mixed.

3. Place a nonstick griddle or skillet over medium heat and let it get hot. Spoon two tablespoons of batter to form a pancake on the griddle. Fry on one side until it starts to bubble, then flip to cook the other side. Cook the entire batch.

4. Serve with low sugar preserves, sugar-free syrup, and butter.

White Bread

Makes: 20 slices

Ingredients:

- 2 cups water
- 1/2 cup oat bran
- 4 Tbsp psyllium husks
- 1 1/2 cup vital wheat gluten
- 1 cup vanilla flavored whey protein powder

- 3/4 cup rice protein powder
- 2 tsp salt
- 2 Tbsp oil
- 2 Tbsp Splenda
- 4 Tbsp yeast

Instructions:

2. Pour all of the ingredients into a bread machine and process based on the manufacturer's instructions.

3. Remove the loaf and set aside to cool.

Peach and Sour Cream Muffins

Makes: 6 large muffins

Ingredients:

- 1/2 cup of soy flour
- 1/2 cup of vanilla protein powder
- 1/2 tsp baking powder
- 1/4 tsp salt
- 1/4 tsp baking soda
- 1 Tbsp Stevia-FOS blend
- 1/2 cup sour cream
- 1/4 cup melted butter

- 1 Tbsp cream
- 2 eggs
- 1 tsp orange peel
- 3/4 cup slightly thawed and diced frozen peaches

Instructions:

1. Preheat oven to 350°F (180°C).

2. In a mixing bowl, combine the dry ingredients in a small bowl.

3. In a separate bowl, combine the butter, cream, sour cream, egg, and orange peel.

4. Add the peaches to the dry ingredients then combine the dry with the wet ingredients. Mix until well distributed.

5. Line a muffin tin with paper cups and spoon your batter to fill the tin. Bake for 20 to 25 minutes.

Low Carb Recipes for Weight Loss

CHAPTER 2

10 LOW CARB LUNCH AND DINNER RECIPES

Grilled Chicken Salad

Makes: 2 servings

Ingredients:

- 3/4 lb boneless, skinless chicken breast
- 2 cups iceberg lettuce, chopped
- 2 cups chopped leaf lettuce
- 3/4 cup chopped red cabbage
- 1/6 cup canned pineapple chunks in juice, diced into small pieces
- 1/4 cup salsa
- 3 Tbsp Teriyaki sauce
- Lime and Mustard Dressing

Teriyaki Sauce:

- 1/4 cup soy sauce
- 1/8 cup dry sherry

- 1 clove garlic, crushed
- 1 Tbsp Splenda
- 1/2 Tbsp grated fresh ginger root

Lime and Mustard Dressing:

- 1/8 cup Dijon mustard
- 1/8 cup Splenda
- 3/4 Tbsp maple syrup
- 3/4 Tbsp canola oil
- 3/4 Tbsp cider vinegar
- 3/4 Tbsp lime juice

Instructions:

Teriyaki Sauce:

Mix all of the ingredients together in a bowl.

Honey Lime and Mustard Dressing:

In a bowl, whisk all of the ingredients together.

Grilled Chicken Salad:

1. Marinate the chicken in the Teriyaki sauce inside the refrigerator for at least 2 hours and preferably overnight.

2. In a salad bowl, combine the iceberg and leaf lettuces, red cabbage, and pineapple bits.

3. Prepare your chicken for grilling by draining the marinade into a bowl and grilling the chicken, basting it with the marinade. Cook on both sides for 3 to 5 minutes or until well done. Slice cooked chicken into pieces.

4. Toss the salad with the Lime and Mustard Dressing. Distribute salad between two plates and top with sliced grilled chicken. Spoon salsa on top of the chicken and serve.

Salmon Patties

Makes: 4 servings

Ingredients:

- 8 oz salmon
- 1/8 cup oat bran
- 1/2 beaten egg
- 1 scallion, finely sliced
- 1 1/2 Tbsp butter

Instructions:

1. Drain the salmon and mash it in a mixing bowl.

2. Add the egg, oat bran, and scallions. Mix well and form 6 to 8 patties.

3. Place a heavy skillet over medium heat and melt the butter. Saute the salmon patties, making sure to turn once and carefully. Cook for 7 minutes per side or until golden.

Garlic Butter Steak

Makes: 2 servings

Ingredients:

- 2 Tbsp softened butter
- 1 clove garlic, crushed
- 1 1/4 lb steak

Instructions:

1. Combine the butter and garlic in a blender or food processor. Blend well.

2. Grill or broil your steak the way you like it. Spoon the garlic butter on top before serving.

Scallops Vinaigrette

Makes: 4 servings

Ingredients:

- 4 Tbsp minced onion
- 1 red bell pepper, cut into thin strips
- 2 Tbsp olive oil
- 4 cups bay scallops
- 1/4 cup Italian salad dressing
- Guar or xanthan

Instructions:

1. Place a large skillet over medium heat. Pour the olive oil and saute the pepper and onion. Add the scallops and saute until white.

2. Add the salad dressing and stir to coat. Let simmer for 3 to 5 minutes until you get the desired thickness. Serve with a cauliflower dish if desired.

Mexiburgers

Makes: 2 servings

Ingredients:

- 2 hamburger patties
- 2 oz jalapeno Monterey Jack cheese
- 2 Tbsp salsa

Instructions:

1. Cook the burger the way you like it. Melt the cheese on top.

2. Spoon the salsa on top and serve with a salad.

Chicken Continental

Makes: 8 servings

Ingredients:

- 2 lb boneless chicken breasts, pounded thin
- 1/2 lb ham, thinly sliced
- 1 lb Asiago cheese, thinly sliced

Instructions:

1. Preheat oven 375 degrees F (190 degrees C).

2. Spread the layer of chicken, followed by ham and cheese in a stoneware pan or casserole. The cheese should completely cover the meats to preserve the juices.

3. Bake for 25 minutes or until cheese becomes golden brown. Serve immediately.

Baked Orange Roughy

Makes: 2 servings

Ingredients:

- 3/4 lb orange roughy fillets, cut into serving size pieces
- 1/2 tsp salt
- Pepper
- 1/2 tsp medium onion, thinly sliced
- Juice of 1/2 lemon or 1 Tbsp lemon juice
- 1/8 cup melted butter
- Paprika
- Optional: minced fresh parsley

Instructions:

1. Preheat oven to 325 degrees F.

2. Grease a shallow baking dish. Place the fish in the pan in a single

layer. Season with salt and pepper. Top with onion.

3. In a bowl, mix the butter and lemon juice, then pour this over the fish. Season with paprika.

4. Bake for 30 minutes, uncovered. Add parsley on top if desired.

Pork Chops

Makes: 3 servings

Ingredients:

- 3 pork chops
- 4 Tbsp soy sauce
- Celery salt
- Garlic powder
- 1/8 cup lemon juice

Instructions:

1. Place the chops on a platter and pour soy sauce and lemon juice on top. Sprinkle with celery salt and garlic powder. Turn and season on the other side.

2. Broil or grill the pork chops the way you like it for at least 5 minutes per side. Baste with any remaining sauce as you do so to keep the chops juicy. Serve.

"Stick-less" Satay

Makes: 2 servings

Ingredients:

- 2 Tbsp oil
- 2 clove garlic, crushed
- 2 tsp curry powder
- 2 boneless, skinless chicken breasts
- Peanut Sauce

Peanut Sauce:

- 1/4 tsp peeled and thinly sliced fresh ginger
- 1/4 cup natural peanut butter, creamy
- 1/4 cup chicken broth
- 1/4 tsp lemon juice
- 1/4 tsp soy sauce
- A few drops of Tabasco sauce
- 1 small clove garlic, crushed
- 1/4 tsp Splenda

Instructions:

1. To make the peanut sauce: Blend all of the peanut sauce ingredients in a blender until smooth.

2. Place a heavy skillet over medium heat. Pour the oil and saute the garlic and curry powder. Add the chicken breasts and saute for 7 minutes per side or until done.

3. Serve with warm peanut sauce.

Aioli Fish Bake

Makes: 2 servings

Ingredients:

- 2 fillets mild white fish
- 2 Tbsp grated Parmesan cheese
- 4 Tbsp Aioli

Aioli:

- 1 clove garlic, crushed
- 1/2 beaten egg
- 1/8 tsp salt
- 1/2 Tbsp lemon juice
- 1/4 cup olive oil

Instructions:

1. To make the Aioli: Place the egg, salt, lemon juice, and garlic in a blender. Blend to combine while gradually pouring the oil into it. Once the sauce becomes thick, turn off the blender.

2. Preheat oven to 350 degrees F (120 degrees C).

3. Grease a baking pan and place the fillets in it. Spread the Aioli on the fillets and top with Parmesan cheese. Turn and spread some more Aioli and sprinkle more Parmesan.

4. Bake for 20 minutes and serve.

CHAPTER 3

10 LOW CARB SIDE DISH RECIPES

Grilled Asparagus and Balsamic Vinegar

Makes: 6 servings

Ingredients:

- 2 lb asparagus
- 4 Tbsp olive oil
- 4 Tbsp balsamic vinegar
- 6 Tbsp grated Parmesan cheese

Instructions:

1. Remove the asparagus ends and drizzle the asparagus with olive oil. Toss to coat. Grill until tender with brown spots. Keep warm by storing in a lidded glass dish.

2. Drizzle balsamic vinegar on top and toss to coat. Sprinkle with Parmesan cheese and serve.

Dilled Beans

Makes: 4 servings

Ingredients:

- 1/2 lb frozen crosscut green beans
- 1/4 cup wine vinegar
- 1/4 cup water
- 1 clove garlic
- 1 tsp salt
- 1 tsp red pepper flakes
- 1 1/2 Tbsp dried dill weed

Instructions:

1. Steam the beans until al dente.

2. In the meantime, mix the water, vinegar, garlic, flakes, dill, salt, and pepper in a saucepan. Place over medium heat and bring to a boil.

3. Drain the beans and place them into a jar with a tight lid. Pour the vinegar mixture over the beans and cover. Refrigerate for at least 24 hours, making sure to shake the jar as often as possible. Serve cold.

Stir-fried Green Beans with Water Chestnuts

Makes: 6 servings

Low Carb Recipes for Weight Loss

Ingredients:

- 4 Tbsp oil
- 4 cups frozen green beans, thawed
- 1 cup drained, sliced or diced canned water chestnuts
- 2 cloves garlic, crushed
- 1/2 cup chicken broth
- 3 tsp soy sauce
- Xanthan or guar

Instructions:

1. Place a wok or skillet over high heat and heat the oil. Saute the green beans and water chestnuts until green beans become tender yet al dente.

2. Add the garlic, soy sauce, and chicken broth. Bring to a simmer and add the xanthan or gum. Stir and let juices thicken, then remove from heat and serve.

Cucumber Salad

Makes: 4 servings

Ingredients:

- 3 small cucumbers, thinly sliced
- 1 1/2 tsp salt
- 1/8 cup Splenda

- 1/8 cup vinegar
- 1/2 cup sour cream
- 1/4 cup finely chopped onion
- 1/2 tsp chopped fresh dill weed
- Salt
- Pepper

Instructions:

1. Place the cucumbers in a large bowl and season with salt. Refrigerate for 2 hours.

2. Drain any excess liquid from the cucumbers. Rinse and drain.

3. In a bowl, combine the Splenda with vinegar until it dissolves, then add the sour cream, dill, and onion. Fold with the cucumbers. Season with salt to taste and serve.

Cauliflower and Cheese Salad

Makes: 3 to 4 servings

Ingredients:

- 1/2 head cauliflower
- 1/8 cup mayonnaise
- 4 oz cream cheese
- 8 oz sour cream
- 1/4 tsp salt

- 1/4 tsp pepper
- 1/4 tsp garlic powder
- 1 cup shredded cheddar cheese
- 1/4 cup onion

Instructions:

1. Slice the cauliflower into bite sized florets. Rinse and drain thoroughly.

2. In a mixing bowl, mix the mayonnaise and cream cheese with an electric beater until smooth. Add sour cream, garlic powder, salt, and pepper. Mix well.

3. In a separate bowl, mix together the cauliflower, onion, and shredded cheddar. Pour the dressing over the cauliflower and fold to combine. Serve.

Tomatoes Basilico

Makes: 2 servings

Ingredients:

- 2 medium size ripe tomatoes
- 1/4 cup fresh, coarsely chopped basil

Instructions:

1. Slice the tomatoes and place them on a platter.

2. Sprinkle with chopped basil and let stand for at least 30 minutes before serving.

Brussels Sprouts and Browned Butter

Makes: 3 to 4 servings

Ingredients:

- 1/2 lb fresh Brussels sprouts, cleaned and trimmed
- 4 Tbsp butter
- Zest of 1/4 lemon
- Juice of 1/2 lemon
- Salt
- Pepper

Instructions:

1. Process Brussels sprouts with the slicing blade of a food processor.

2. In a heavy skillet, melt the butter until brown. Add the Brussels sprouts, lemon zest and juice and saute until al dente. Season with salt and pepper. Serve.

Aragula and Pear Salad

Makes: 4 servings

Ingredients:

- 8 cups washed, dried, and torn up aragula

- 1 ripe pear, cut into small chunks
- 6 Tbsp extra virgin olive oil
- Juice of 2 lemons
- Salt
- Pepper
- 4 Tbsp finely sliced Parmesan cheese

Instructions:

1. In a salad bowl, toss the aragula and pear to combine. Add olive oil and toss.

2. Add lemon juice and season with salt and pepper, toss. Top with Parmesan and serve.

Roasted Cabbage and Balsamic Vinegar

Makes: 3 to 4 servings

Ingredients:

- 1/4 head red cabbage
- 1/4 head cabbage
- 1 1/2 Tbsp olive oil
- Salt
- Pepper
- 1 Tbsp balsamic vinegar

Instructions:

1. Preheat oven to 450 degrees F (230 degrees C).

2. Chop the cabbages coarsely. Strew over a roasting pan and drizzle with olive oil. Toss to coat. Season with salt and pepper and toss to combine.

3. Roast cabbages for 15 minutes, stirring once. Remove from oven once leaves have browned around the edges, but still crisp. Drizzle with balsamic vinegar, toss, and serve.

Broccoli and Cashew Salad

Makes: 4 servings

Ingredients:

- 1 Tbsp cider vinegar
- 1/8 cup Splenda
- 1/2 cup mayo
- 1 small bunch broccoli
- 1 cup red seedless grapes
- 1/4 purple onion, chopped
- 1/2 lb bacon, cooked to a crisp and chopped
- 1/2 cup roasted, salted cashews

Instructions:

1. Place cider vinegar in a microwaveable bowl and whisk in the Splenda. Heat in microwave for a few seconds until Splenda has melted. Add the mayo and mix to combine. Set aside.

2. Chop the broccoli into the same size as the grapes. Slice the grapes in half and mix together with the broccoli. Add the onion and crumble the bacon into the mixture. Toss to mix.

3. Pour the dressing over the salad and toss to coat. Sprinkle the cashews on top and toss to distribute. Serve.

CHAPTER 4

10 LOW CARB SNACK RECIPES

Soy and Ginger Pecans

Makes: 4 servings

Ingredients:

- 1 cup shelled pecans
- 2 Tbsp melted butter
- 1 1/2 Tbsp soy sauce
- 1/2 tsp ground ginger

Instructions:

1. Preheat oven to 300 degrees F (148 degrees C)

2. Strew the pecans across a shallow roasting pan. Add the butter and stir to coat. Roast for 15 minutes.

3. Remove from heat and add the soy sauce. Stir to coat. Sprinkle the ginger on top and stir to coat as well. Roast for 10 more minutes then set aside to cool before serving.

Cajun Trail Mix

Makes: 1 1/2 cups

Ingredients:

- 1/2 cup dry roasted peanuts
- 1/2 cup raw cashew pieces
- 1/2 cup pecans
- 1/4 cup low-sugar raisins
- 2 Tbsp low-fat butter
- 1/2 tsp paprika
- 1/4 tsp garlic powder
- 1/4 tsp onion powder
- 1/8 tsp cayenne
- 1/8 tsp dried oregano
- 1/8 tsp dried thyme
- 1/8 tsp pepper
- 1/2 tsp Worcestershire sauce
- Salt to taste

Instructions:

1. Toss the peanuts, cashews, and pecans in a baking pan.

2. Melt the butter and combine the garlic and onion powders, cayenne, dried oregano and thyme, pepper, and Worcestershire sauce. Pour

this over the mixed nuts, making sure to spoon out any remaining seasoning from the bottom. Stir to coat.

3. Roast the mixed nuts at 300 degrees F (150 degrees C) for 30 minutes. Stir the nuts after the first 15 minutes. Season with salt to taste and toss in the raisins.

Saganaki

Makes: 4 servings

Ingredients:

- 1/2 lb Kasseri, in a 1/2 inch thick slab
- 2 eggs, beaten
- 4 to 5 Tbsp rice protein or soy powder
- Olive oil
- 2 shots brandy
- 1/2 lemon

Instructions:

1. Dip the cheese in the beaten egg, then dip it in the protein or soy powder to coat.

2. Place a heavy skillet over medium heat and heat about 1/4 inch of olive oil. Let it heat up, then add the cheese.

3. Fry until it becomes crisp and golden, turning just once. Place onto a heat resistant plate.

4. Pour the brandy on top of the hot cheese and light it up with a match.

5. Squeeze the lemon over the flame to put out the fire and slice, then serve.

Cheese Cookies

Makes: 3 dozen small cookies

Ingredients:

- 1/4 lb processed American loaf cheese
- 1/4 lb sharp Cheddar cheese
- 1/8 lb butter
- 1/2 cup soy powder
- Optional: 3 dozen walnut or pecan halves

Instructions:

1. Preheat oven to 400 degrees F (204 degrees C).

2. Slice the loaf cheese, Cheddar, and butter into chunks. Put them in a food processor. Add the soy powder and pulse until thoroughly mixed.

3. Grease a cookie sheet and put spoonfuls of dough on top. Press half a walnut or pecan on top, if desired. Bake for 8 minutes or until cookies become brown around the edges.

Tuna Stuffed Eggs

Makes: 6 servings

Ingredients:

- 6 hard-boiled free range eggs
- 1 1/2 oz canned tuna, drained
- 1/8 cup mayonnaise
- 1 small red onion, finely minced
- 2 stalks celery, finely minced
- 1/4 tsp chili garlic paste
- 1/2 tsp prepared horseradish
- 1/2 tsp grated Parmesan cheese

Instructions:

1. Slice the eggs in half and spoon the yolks out and place them into a medium size bowl. Place the whites on a serving plate.

2. Combine the mayonnaise and tuna with the egg yolks with a fork, mashing them until everything is combined thoroughly.

3. Add the minced red onion and celery to the mixture. Add the horseradish and garlic paste. Mix well.

4. Stuff the whites with the tuna mixture, distributing it evenly. Top with Parmesan cheese and serve.

Low Carb Recipes for Weight Loss

Hot Wings

Makes: 12 pieces

Ingredients:

- 1/2 tsp cayenne pepper
- 1 tsp dried oregano
- 1/2 tsp curry powder
- 1 tsp paprika
- 1 tsp dried thyme
- 1 lb chicken wings, cut into drumettes

Instructions:

1. Preheat oven to 375 degrees F (190 degrees C).

2. In a bowl, mix the oregano, pepper, curry, thyme, and paprika.

3. Place the chicken wings in a shallow baking pan and sprinkle the seasoning mix on top. Coat evenly on both sides.

4. Roast for 45 minutes or until crisp. Serve with blue cheese dressing, if desired.

Brie and Walnut Quesadillas

Makes: 3 to 4 servings

Ingredients:

- 1/5 cup chopped walnuts

- 5 oz Brie
- 4 low carb tortillas

Instructions:

1. Preheat oven to 350 degrees F (180 degrees C).

2. Strew walnuts in a shallow roasting pan and roast for 8 minutes.

3. In the meantime, slice the Brie into quarters, making sure to slice off the rind. Cut Brie into cubes.

4. Place a heavy skillet over medium-low heat and heat a tortilla, then cover it with pieces of Brie and let the heat melt the cheese.

5. Remove the walnuts from the oven and strew a few walnuts over the cheese. Top with another tortilla and turn it over to cook the other side. Transfer to a plate and cover to keep warm. Repeat with the second batch.

6. Slice into wedges and serve.

Pizza Muffin Bites

Makes: 15 pieces

Ingredients:

- 1 Tbsp olive oil
- 1 clove garlic, minced
- 1/4 cup chopped green pepper
- 1/4 cup chopped red pepper

Low Carb Recipes for Weight Loss

- 1/4 small onion, chopped
- 1/2 cup chopped mushrooms
- 1/8 cup chopped olives
- 1/4 tsp red pepper flakes
- 1/4 tsp Italian seasoning
- Black pepper to taste
- 1 egg
- 3/4 cup shredded mozzarella
- 1/3 cup grated Parmesan cheese
- 4 oz cream cheese
- 15 slices of deli-sized pepperoni
- 1/4 cup pizza sauce

Instructions:

1. Place a skillet over medium heat and pour the olive oil. Saute the garlic, onion, and peppers for 1 minute. Add the mushrooms and saute for 2 minutes. Remove from heat and stir in the olives. Season with red pepper flakes, black pepper, and Italian seasoning.

2. In a mixing bowl, whisk the eggs and add the mozzarella, Parmesan, and cream cheese. Pour the sauteed garlic, onion, and peppers into the mixture and whisk to combine.

3. Prepare a mini-muffin cup and place a slice of pepperoni inside to serve as the "crust". With a teaspoon, put some of the cheese and vegetable mixture into each cup. B

4. Bake for 25 minutes at 325 degrees F (170 degrees C). 10 minutes before the end of cooking time, pour a bit of pizza sauce on top. Serve warm.

Indian Punks

Makes: 2 servings

Ingredients:

- 2 Tbsp butter
- 1 1/4 Tbsp curry powder
- 1 clove garlic, crushed
- 1 cup raw, shelled pumpkin seeds
- Salt

Instructions:

1. Preheat oven to 300 degrees F (148 degrees C).

2. Place a small skillet over medium heat and melt the butter. Add the garlic and curry powder. Stir for 2 minutes.

3. Put the pumpkin seeds in a bowl and pour the butter on top. Stir to coat.

4. Spread the mixture in a shallow roasting pan and roast for 25 minutes. Season lightly with salt.

Low Carb Recipes for Weight Loss

Spinach Stuffed Mushrooms

Makes: 20 pieces

Ingredients:

- 3/4 lb mushrooms, cleaned and wiped dry
- 1 Tbsp low-fat butter
- 1/4 cup chopped onion
- 2 cloves garlic, crushed
- 5 oz frozen chopped spinach, thawed
- 2 oz cream cheese
- 1/8 tsp pepper
- 1/4 tsp salt
- 3/4 tsp Worcestershire sauce
- 1/8 cup Parmesan cheese

Instructions:

1. Preheat oven to 350 degrees F (180 degrees C).

2. Remove the stems from the mushrooms and finely chop the stems.

3. Place a large heavy-duty skillet over medium-low heat and heat the butter. Sauté the chopped mushroom stems and onions until onions become translucent and the stems change in color. Add the crushed garlic and sauté for 2 minutes.

4. In the meantime, place the thawed spinach into a strainer and squeeze as much of the liquid out as possible. Add spinach to the onion and mushroom mixture. Add the cream cheese and stir until it melts.

Season with salt & pepper, Worcestershire sauce, and Parmesan.

5. Spoon the spinach and mushroom mixture into the mushroom caps. Place them on a baking pan. Sprinkle any remaining Parmesan cheese on top. Pour just enough water to cover the base of the pan and prevent the mushrooms from being overcooked.

6. Bake for 25 to 30 minutes and serve immediately.

CHAPTER 5

10 LOW CARB DESSERT RECIPES

Butter Pecan Bites

Makes: 8 bars

Ingredients:

- 1/2 stick salted butter
- 1/2 Tbsp molasses
- 1/2 cup Splenda
- 1 egg
- 1/4 tsp vanilla
- 1/8 cup almond meal
- 1/8 cup oat flour or 1/4 cup low-carb flour
- 1/2 cup chopped pecans

Instructions:

1. Preheat oven to 325 degrees F (170 degrees C).
2. Place the butter in a microwaveable bowl and melt it in the

microwave on 40 percent power for 1 minute. Add the molasses, Splenda, eggs, and vanilla. Stir to combine. Add the almond meal and oat or low-carb flour. Stir to combine. Add the pecans and stir to distribute evenly.

3. Grease a baking pan or mini-muffin pan with oil and transfer the batter into it. Bake for 25 minutes.

Coconut Shortbread

Makes: 2 dozen cookies

Ingredients:

- 1/4 cup butter, at room temperature
- 1/4 cup coconut oil
- 1 1/2 Tbsp Splenda
- 3/4 cup vanilla flavored whey protein powder
- 1/2 cup finely shredded, unsweetened coconut
- 1 Tbsp water

Instructions:

1. Preheat oven to 375 degrees F (190 degrees C).

2. Combine the butter, coconut oil, and Splenda with an electric mixer until creamy. Add the protein powder, coconut, and water, and beat until thoroughly mixed.

3. Line a jelly roll pan with parchment, and transfer the dough into it. Place a second sheet of parchment over the dough and press to even out. Score the dough into small rectangles with a sharp knife. Bake for 7 minutes or until golden brown. Cool and break into pieces.

Brownies

Makes: 6 servings

Ingredients:

- 1 oz bitter chocolate
- 4 oz butter
- 1/4 cup polyol sweetener
- 1/4 cup Splenda
- 1 egg
- 1/4 cup vanilla whey protein powder
- Salt

Instructions:

1. Preheat oven 350 degrees F (180 degrees C).

2. Place a saucepan on top of a double boiler. Place over a heat diffuser set on very low heat. Melt the chocolate and butter in the saucepan and stir to mix well. Transfer into a bowl.

3. Pour the polyol sweetener into the butter and chocolate mixture. Stir to combine. Add the Splenda and stir. Add the egg and whisk well. Add the vanilla whey protein powder and a sparse pinch of salt. Stir well.

4. Grease a baking pan and pour the batter into it. Bake for 15 minutes. Cut into bars and set aside to cool.

Cocoa Peanut Logs

Makes: approximately 18 logs

Ingredients:

- 3 oz sugar free chocolate bars or chips
- 1/4 cup natural peanut butter, salted
- 2 cups crisp soy cereal

Instructions:

1. Place a double boiler or heat diffuser over very low heat and melt the chocolate and peanut butter together. Mix well. Add the cereal and stir until well coated.

2. Grease a baking pan and line with foil. Transfer the cereal mixture onto the pan and chill for at least 3 hours. Slice into squares and keep chilled until ready to serve.

Blueberry Cobbler

Makes: 5 servings

Ingredients:

- 2 cups fresh or unsweetened frozen blueberries
- 1/8 cup Splenda
- 1/8 cup polyol sweetener
- 1/2 Tbsp lemon juice
- 4 Tbsp butter
- 1/4 cup almond meal

Low Carb Recipes for Weight Loss

- 1/4 cup vanilla whey protein powder
- 1 1/4 tsp baking powder
- 1/2 Tbsp Splenda
- 1 tsp salt
- 1/4 cup heavy cream

Instructions:

1. Preheat oven to 275 degrees F (190 degrees C). Grease a baking pan and set aside.

2. In a bowl, mix the blueberries together with 1/8 cup Splenda, polyol sweetener, and lemon juice. Toss to coat and transfer into the pan. Distribute evenly. Spoon two 1/2 tablespoons of butter.

3. In a bowl, mix together the almond meal, 1/2 tablespoon Splenda, vanilla whey, baking powder, and salt.

4. Melt 3 tablespoons of butter and combine with the cream in a bowl. Add this to the dry ingredients stir well until thoroughly mixed.

5. Pour the batter over the blueberries in the pan, making sure it is even. Bake for 30 minutes or until the crust is golden brown. Serve warm.

Eggnog Ice Cream

Makes: 2 servings

Ingredients:

- 1/2 package unflavored and unsweetened gelatin
- 1/2 cup hot water

- 1/2 tsp vanilla extract
- Optional: 1/2 tsp brandy extract
- 3/4 cup heavy cream
- 1/6 cup Splenda
- 1/8 tsp nutmeg
- 1/8 tsp cinnamon
- 1/4 tsp liquid sweetener
- 1/8 cup egg white protein

Instructions:

1. Gradually pour the gelatin into the hot water and let stand for 1 minute. Stir until dissolved.

2. Put the vanilla and brandy extracts (if using), heavy cream, Splenda, cinnamon, nutmeg, liquid sweetener, prepared gelatin, and egg protein in a food processor or blender. Blend until thoroughly combined.

3. Chill for at least 30 minutes, then stir and pour into an ice cream maker. Follow the manufacturer's instructions.

Cherry Cheesecake

Makes: 6 servings

Ingredients:

- 1 lb cream cheese, softened
- 1 1/2 Tbsp Splenda

Low Carb Recipes for Weight Loss

- 1/2 tsp vanilla
- 1 cup whipped cream
- Sugarless Cherry Pie filling

Sugarless Cherry Pie Filling:

- 7 oz sour cherries in water
- 1/4 cup Splenda
- 1 tsp xanthan or guar
- Optional: red food coloring

Instructions:

1. To make the cherry pie filling: In a bowl, mix the cherries in water (together with the water), Splenda, and xanthan or guar. If using food coloring, add 2 to 4 drops. Set aside for 5 minutes before serving.

2. Put the cream cheese, Splenda, vanilla, and whipped cream in a mixer and mix until thoroughly combined. Pour the mixture into a glass dish and spoon the cherry pie filling on top. Serve chilled.

Fudge Toffee

Makes: approximately 18 squares

Ingredients:

- 1 cup Splenda
- 1/2 cup whole milk powder

Low Carb Diet For Weight Loss Secrets

- 1/2 cup natural whey protein powder
- 1/4 cup melted unsalted butter
- 1/8 cup whipped cream
- 1 Tbsp water
- 1 oz unsweetened baking chocolate, melted

Instructions:

1. In a mixing bowl, mix together the milk powder, Splenda, and protein powder.

2. In a separate bowl, mix together the cream, butter, and water. Add this to the dry ingredients. Add the melted chocolate and stir to combine.

3. Transfer the mixture into a baking dish. Freeze for at least half and hour, then refrigerate. Cut into squares and serve.

Strawberry Daiquiris

Makes: 2 to 3 servings

Ingredients:

- 2 cups fresh or frozen and thawed unsweetened strawberries
- 1/4 cup light rum
- 1/8 cup lime juice
- 1/8 cup Splenda
- 2 cups crushed ice

Instructions:

1. Put the strawberries, lime juice, rum, and Splenda in a blender. Blend until smooth. Add the crushed ice and blend until thoroughly mixed.

Sesame Cookies

Makes: approximately 30 cookies

Ingredients:

- 1/4 cup butter
- 1/2 cup Splenda
- 1/2 beaten egg
- 1/2 cup tahini
- 1/4 tsp salt
- 1/4 tsp baking soda
- 3/4 cup vanilla flavored whey protein powder
- 1/8 cup sesame seeds

Instructions:

1. Preheat oven to 375 degrees F (190 degrees C).

2. Beat the butter and Splenda with an electric beater until smooth. Add the egg and beat, then the tahini and beat once more.

3. Add baking soda and salt, then add the protein powder. Beat well to mix. Add the sesame seeds and stir until well distributed.

4. Grease a cookie sheet and drop tablespoonfuls of dough. Bake for 10 minutes or until golden.

Low Carb Recipes for Weight Loss

CONCLUSION

Thank you again for buying this book!

I hope this book was able to help you to make low carb recipes at home.

The next step is to create a consistent low carb meal plan and stick to it so that you can attain your weight loss goal.

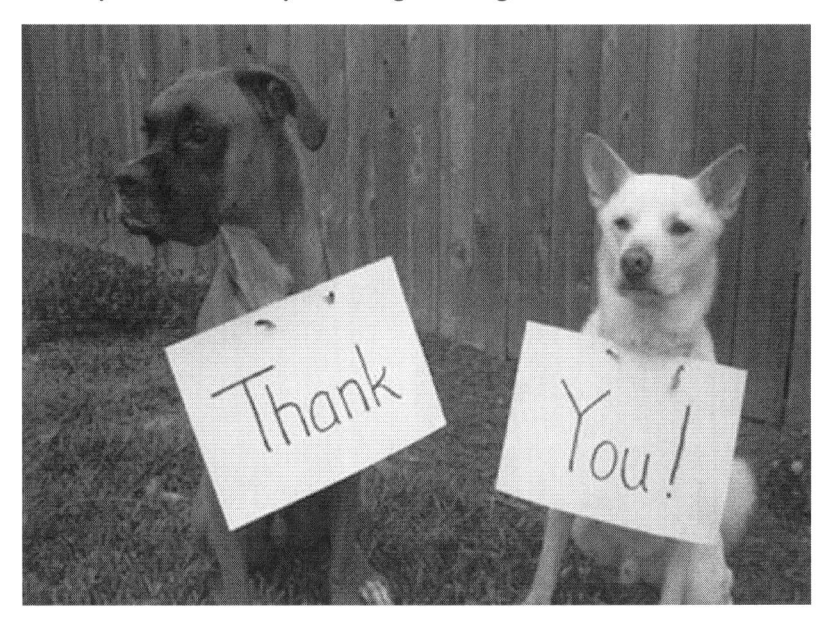

Finally, if you enjoyed this book, then I'd like to ask you for a favor, would you be kind enough to leave a review for this book on Amazon? It'd be greatly appreciated!

Thank you and good luck!